Prof. Arnold Ehret's

PHYSICAL FITNESS THRU A SUPERIOR DIET, FASTING, AND DIETETICS

ALSO

A RELIGIOUS CONCEPT OF PHYSICAL, SPIRITUAL, AND MENTAL DIETETICS

Introduced & Edited by Prof. Spira

PROF. ARNOLD EHRET'S

PHYSICAL FITNESS THRU A SUPERIOR DIET

FASTING, AND DIETETICS

ALSO

A RELIGIOUS CONCEPT OF PHYSICAL, SPIRITUAL, AND

MENTAL DIETETICS

By Prof. Arnold Ehret (1866-1922)

Introduced & Edited by Prof. Spira

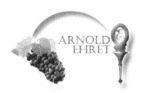

Published by Breathair Publishing

Columbus, OH

1st Edition 2018

Printed by CreateSpace, an Amazon.com Company
CreateSpace, Charleston SC

Available from www.mucusfreelife.com, Amazon.com, on Kindle, and other retail outlets

Printed in the United States of America

First Printing, 2018
First Edition

ISBN-13: 978-0-9977026-4-4
ISBN-10: 0-9977026-4-8

www.mucusfreelife.com

Discover other titles by Breathair Publishing

Prof. Arnold Ehret's Mucusless Diet Healing System: Annotated, Revised, and Edited by Prof. Spira

Spira Speaks: Dialogs and Essays on the Mucusless Diet Healing System

Prof. Arnold Ehret's Rational Fasting for Physical, Mental and Spiritual Rejuvenation: Introduced and Edited by Prof. Spira

Thus Speaketh the Stomach and the Tragedy of Nutrition: Introduced and Edited by Prof. Spira

The Definite Cure of Chronic Constipation and Overcoming Constipation Naturally: Introduced and Edited by Prof. Spira

Coming Soon

Mucusless Diet Healing System eCourse: Keys for Mastering a Mucus-free Life

Contents

Introduction by Prof. Spira

Greetings Brothers and Sisters,

Physical Fitness Thru a Superior Diet, Fasting, and Dietetics Also a Religious Concept of Physical, Spiritual, and Mental Dietetics include articles by Prof. Arnold Ehret, originator of the *Mucusless Diet Healing System*, which philosophically explore humanity's potential to manifest paradise on Earth through mucus-free living, rational fasting, and physical fitness.

Fred S. Hirsch (1888–1979), former owner of Ehret Literature Publishing and close friend of Ehret, published a compilation of Ehret's works entitled *Physical Culture: Fasting & Dietetics, The Exact Diagnosis of Your Disease, The Magic Mirror* in 1938. This release includes Ehret's article "Physical Culture," compiled with some of Ehret's other writings. Historically, the term "physical culture" refers to a health and strength training movement that originated during the 19th century in Germany, England, and the United States. Following 1848, German immigrants introduced a physical fitness system based on gymnastics that became popular in colleges and public schools. Following the First Industrial Revolution, reformers showed concern for the health of sedentary white-collar workers, and sought to promote diet and exercise as a way to counteract the inactive lifestyles of many members of the burgeoning middle and upper classes.

Before the Industrial Revolution, the term "fitness" referred to the ability for one to complete a day's work without undue fatigue. In the 1950s, however, the use of the term "fitness" increased exponentially in the Western vernacular and came to mean a state of health, well-being, stamina, and strength. In 1966, Fred Hirsch changed the title of "Physical Culture" to "Physical Fitness Thru a Superior Diet, Fasting, & Dietetics" and paired it with Ehret's article "A Religious Concept of Physical, Spiritual, & Mental Dietetics." The latter compilation remained available from Ehret Literature Publishing until the early 2000s. At the time of the release of our edition, there are no others in print and readily available.

Collected in this edition are the two articles compiled in the 1966 release, including "Physical Fitness thru a Superior Diet, Fasting, and Dietetics," and "A Religious Concept of Physical, Spiritual, and Mental Dietetics." In the former, Arnold Ehret contributes his conception of how humans can learn to live a natural life through a historical dialogue that fits within the Western philosophical tradition. In the latter, Ehret's message is directed toward spiritual and religious readers as he shares ideas surrounding his theological philosophy of "Physiological Christianism." In both articles, I fixed typographical errors from the original text and made minor changes to outdated gender-specific terminology or language considered insensitive and politically incorrect by today's standards. As the editor, my aim is not to change Ehret's work, but make this document as accessible as possible to contemporary readers.

Additional writings include the "Biographical Sketch of Prof. Arnold Ehret" by B.W. Child, and Ehret's "The Enforcement of Elimination by Physical Adjustments, Exercises, Sunbaths, Internal Baths, and Bathing," and "A Message to Ehretists." The biographical sketch, which first appeared in the 1924 edition of *Prof. Arnold Ehret's Mucusless Diet Healing System*, fits well amongst the thought-provoking articles in this compilation. It provides an illuminating testimonial by Ehret on his journey to heal himself of an "incurable" disease, and how he discovered the keys to regenerating the human body, mind, and spirit.

The final two writings are from the annotated, edited, and revised edition of the *Mucusless Diet Healing System*. "The Enforcement of

Elimination by Physical Adjustments, Exercises, Internal Baths, and Bathing" is Lesson XXV from the *Mucusless Diet*. In this lesson, Ehret explores auxiliary therapies to his dietary methods, including exercise, sunbathing, internal baths (enemas), and external baths. Finally, "A Message to Ehretists" is Ehret's conclusion to the *Mucusless Diet Healing System* where he clarifies fundamentals of his back-to-nature philosophy and encourages the reader to join his movement toward a disease-free paradise on Earth. Both of these writings pair well with the philosophical discussions about physical health and spiritual well-being found in the first two articles.

I strongly encourage you to read this book along with Arnold Ehret's other works, including the *Mucusless Diet Healing System, Rational Fasting, Definite Cure of Chronic Constipation,* and *Thus Speaketh the Stomach*. Perhaps most important is Ehret's *Mucusless Diet Healings System,* which provides an in-depth and comprehensive look at Ehret's important philosophical contributions as well as practical instructions to apply his acclaimed *Healing System.*

Ehret's message of hope for humanity is needed today more than ever. Humans are destroying themselves and the Earth on an unprecedented level. Ehret shares his solution for the problems of humanity through his message of superior natural healing. He believes that the source of all problems in the world is an improper and unnatural diet. Thus, the dysfunction of governments, police brutality, war, the mistreatment of the environment, racism, sexism, all forms of bigotry, the disregard for the lives of animals, etc., are all symptoms of a pus- and mucus-laden diet that renders humanity unempathetic and impotent.

How badly do we want to experience paradise? Are we content to live in ignorance and blame everything but diet? Is it easier to continue to believe the propaganda we have been fed? That we need to stuff ourselves with protein and fat? That we must eat certain nutritious foods, although we know that they cause illness? Ehret challenges us to shift our paradigm away from the mucus-based status quo and medical extremism of the 21st century and embrace our true nature as mucus-free beings.

Peace, Love, and Breath!

–Prof. Spira, May 2018

Biographical Sketch of Prof. Arnold Ehret by Prof. B.W. Child

I knew Professor Ehret first as an author, later as a sanitarium proprietor and lecturer, and now esteem him highly as a friend and the pioneer of the most complete natural and scientific system for the Cure and Prevention of Disease known. I have no hesitancy in stating that he has evolved and developed what now seems to be the "last word" in regard to health and longevity.

He was born July 25, 1866, near Freiburg, in Baden, Germany, and lived to be 56 years of age, and was endowed by his father with a natural bent or extraordinary desire for delving into the causes and reasons for occurrences and results.

Ehret's education was obtained at a college where the long walk added to the other work on the farm, on an ordinary diet, brought on a severe attach of bronchial catarrh. In spite of this handicap he graduated with honors. His greatest interest being for physics, chemistry, drawing and painting, he took a special academic course and graduated as professor of drawing for high schools and colleges, at 21 years of age. He taught at a college until drafted for military service, but was released after nine months' service because of "Neurasthenic heart trouble," resuming his vocation as a teacher. At 31 years of age he was quite fleshy and "looked well," as others said, but was suffering from kidney trouble, Bright's disease, with consumptive tendency.

1

In his own words:

"Five times I took vacations to recuperate, but finally was pronounced 'incurable' and resigned. Then for five years I 'suffered much from many physicians' (24 in all) and part of this suffering was to pay the bills of about $6,000, but with the result pronounced 'incurable.' Physically and nearly mentally bankrupt, I thought of suicide, but accidentally heard of naturopathy and was treated at a Kneipp sanitarium three different times, getting some relief and a desire to live, but not cured. Was treated at five or six other Nature Cure sanitariums and tried all other methods known in Europe, expending more thousands, with the result that while not down sick, neither was I healthy. I learned something from the experiences, though; the main symptoms were mucus or pus and albumin in the urine and pain in the kidneys. The doctors, on the presumption that a clear urine indicated health, tried to stop these eliminations with drugs and to replace the albumin by a meat, egg, and milk diet, but it only increased the disastrous results. I reasoned out from these methods what seemed like a great light on the subject, that the right diet should be free from mucus and albumin. My naturopathic treatment drew out some of the mucus by baths, exercise, etc., but fed it back by wrong diet.

"I resolved to face what seemed a tragedy for me (and does now to most chronically sick persons after getting no relief from doctors), and try for myself that which I had learned from past experience: that wrong eating was the *cause* and right eating *might* be the cure. There was vegetarianism, fruit and nut diet, numerous food 'cures' and a few hints that fasting would help. I went to Berlin to study vegetarianism, as there were over twenty vegetarian restaurants there at that time. My first observation was that vegetarians were not much more healthy than meat eaters, for many looked sickly and pale. With the starchy food and milk I grew slowly worse, but started a course of study at the university in medicine, physiology, and chemistry. I visited a school of naturopathy, learned something of mental healing, Christian Science, magnetic healing, etc., etc., all to *try* to find out the real and fundamental truths of perfect health. Was more or less disappointed and went to Nice, in southern France, and tried a radical fruit diet with the exception of a pint of milk a day, thinking then that I needed the albumin. I made no special application of the fruit diet to my condition, as most others did not, and received but little benefit. Some days I felt well and on others felt very bad, so I soon went back home, returning to the so-called 'good eating,' as lived and suggested by well-meaning friends, relatives and physicians. I had learned something about fasting, but it was opposed by all friends and relatives; even my former naturopathic doctor told my sister that to a person with Bright's disease a few days' fast would prove fatal.

"The next winter I went to Algiers, in northern Africa. The mild climate and the wonderful fruits improved my condition and gave me more faith in Nature's methods and an understanding of them, and I gained courage to try short fasts to assist the cleansing properties of fruit and climate, with such results that one morning of a well-feeling day I chanced to notice in my mirror that my face had taken on an entirely new look; that of a younger and healthy looking person. But on the next bad feeling day the old and sickly-looking face returned, yet it did not last long and these alternating changes in my face impressed me as a 'revelation' from Nature that I had found out her methods in part and was on the right track, and I resolved to study them more and live them closer in my future life.

"An indescribable feeling never known before of better health, more vital energy, better efficiency, and more endurance and strength came to me and gave me great joy and happiness just to be alive. This was not only of the physical, but there was a great change in my mental ability to perceive, to remember, greater courage and hope, and above all an insight into the spiritual which became like a sunrise, throwing light upon all higher and spiritual problems. All my faculties were improved, far surpassing their best during my healthiest and best youth. My physical efficiency and endurance became wonderfully increased. I took a bicycle trip of about 800 miles, from Algiers to Tunis, accompanied by a trained bicyclist who lived on an ordinary diet. I was never behind him but often ahead toward night when endurance became the test. Keep in mind that I was formerly a candidate for death, so declared by the doctors, but now jubilant that I could surpass the most efficient, and a constant joy of exhilaration having escaped the 'slaughter house' of humankind, called 'Scientific Medical Clinics.'

3

"Arriving home again, I demonstrated my ability and endurance to perform the hardest farm labor and in tests of strength superior to those in good training on the ordinary diet, but being surrounded by friends and relatives who were living in the ordinary way and coming in contact with professional men who were excited by fear that my discoveries were of true principles and would eventually succeed and surpass those they were practicing, I gradually took up the ordinary diet. Fasting was then very unpopular and living in the family of my sister who threatened to prevent it should I attempt one, I could not take up again what I firmly believed and had proven by actual experience, that fasting (simply eating less) was Nature's Omnipotent method of cleansing the body from the effects of wrong and too much eating. I had also found it the 'Master Key' to mental and spiritual unfoldment and evolution. I had not neglected the study of the scientific reasons *why* fruit and mucusless foods were so efficient, and had found that they developed during the process of digestion what was known as Grape Sugar, and from what was termed carbohydrates by analysis. My experience, tests, and experiments as well as cures, all showed that grape sugar of fruits was the essential material of human food, giving the highest efficiency and endurance, and at the same time was the best eliminator of debris and the most efficient healing agent known for the human body.

"This was in direct contradiction of the nitrogenous-albumin theory of the doctors and scientists and also of the more modern theory of 'mineral salts.' In 1909 I wrote an article denouncing the Metabolic theory and in 1912 learned that Dr. Thomas Powell of Los Angeles had made the same discovery and was making remarkable cures by using foods containing what he called 'organic carbon,' which is the same food ingredients that develop into grape sugar during digestion. With the embryo of these discoveries in mind and my experiences I left my friends and relatives, who would have shortened my life by their well-meaning kindness, and, accompanied by a young man who was won by my experience to try with me experimental diet and fasting for his ailments, the principal one being stuttering, went to southern France. Here, during several months of experiments, I renewed my experiences in Africa and won a firmer belief than ever that fruit diet and fasting were Nature's infallible factors for regaining and maintaining a superior health than is enjoyed by most of civilized humankind.

"The results obtained were often called miraculous, but were only marvelous because of their rareness. The knowledge I had gained of the wonderful methods by which Nature carried on the cleansing from the impurities from wrong food, and then the regenerating, repairing and strengthening, by the *right* food, was the marvel, but not a miracle.

"Especially important were the results on this comparatively young man—ten years younger than I. We made tests with all the general foods of civilization after cleansing fasts. Our now more sensitive organs revolted at once against their undesirable elements and especially against combinations, giving the most convincing evidence that modern cooking, with its mixtures, with but little knowledge of their qualities, was the fundamental cause of all diseases. It is impossible to know what food really is and its effects until the body has been cleansed by Nature's own method, a fast. I have never known of such experiments ever being made by anyone, and the facts gained have now been so abundantly proven during many years of the most searching and difficult practice that they have raised my knowledge above all doubts or arguments about the dietetic opinions of others.

"To test our efficiency at exhaustive labor, we took a trip through northern Italy, walking for 56 hours continuously without sleep or rest or food, only drink. This after a seven-day fast and then only one meal of two pounds of cherries. This was called by the professional minds that knew of it a most marvelous test, from their viewpoint. From what came the energy for this efficiency? From nitrogen, albumin, organic salts, fats, vitamins, or from what? After a 16-hour walk I made a test of knee bendings and arm extendings, 360 times in a few minutes, and later numerous strength tests with athletic competitors showing superior results. These after being pronounced incurable and my father and brother having died of consumption. During our trip through Italy we were often subjects of interesting comments by ladies on our ruddy and healthy complexion and inquiries of how we brought it about, etc. As a completely transformed man, I desired higher experiences, as they were not only physical, but mental and spiritual. The same with my young companion. He was wonderfully improved in many ways, but his stuttering showed no change. I had the idea that even that was caused by a physical encumbrance of debris. We proceeded to a secluded place on the island of Capri and there took longer fasts and daily sunbaths with heat around 120° of four to six hours. We were so well cleansed that we did not sweat. On the eighteenth day my young friend became quite hoarse, and fearing he would lose his voice—not then knowing what caused it—ended his fast with about three pounds of figs, at my suggestion, with the result that for nearly an hour he raised a very large quantity of mucus from his throat and his body cleansed itself in other directions. His voice was soon restored, and his stuttering disappeared and has never returned. We had accomplished what his rich father had in vain tried to do by employing almost every known treatment for him, without the slightest permanent improvement.

"*Fasting*, Nature's Supreme Remedy, has been so crudely practiced, and is so generally misunderstood, that it is very important that it be rightly explained. From my long experience in curing myself by fasting and mucusless diet, and in conducting fasts for many hundreds in my sanitarium in Switzerland, during a period of over ten years, I can state with certainty of its wonderful potency and benefits when rightly conducted. My first experience brought such beneficial results that I desired to perfect and verify the methods employed, so I continued my observations and investigations of and into all phases of life. I made many and very extensive experiments, and then my fully restored young friend and myself started on a long trip. First, through southern Italy, walking and living on an almost exclusive grape diet; then by boat to Egypt, Palestine, Turkey, Rumania and Austria, home. On this trip we learned much of the diet, habits, mentality and health of the different peoples, and especially in the Orient, and with the result that my belief in the superiority of European civilization received a severe shock, and my belief strengthened that I was on the right track for a knowledge of a much superior health with a better mental development, and a more active and longer life.

"In Egypt, we saw a race of people of extraordinary strength and endurance, living on a scanty vegetarian diet mostly, but with two

6

supposedly bad habits—cigarette smoking and drinking strong coffee, yet we saw not a single nervous or toxemic person. To see how few kinds and how little food they ate, to learn that they are about the same kinds of foods that their ancestors ate, gives one a reason for the superior qualities of old Egyptian civilization.

"In Palestine we stayed several months, studying local customs, records and history of past conditions, with the result that my conception of the real meaning of the New Testament gospels was changed very much. I learned that Christ's life and teachings were in strict accord with now well-known natural laws, which brought him superior intelligence and superior health, but that when written up from current hearsay some 150 years after, were colored by oriental forms of expression and metaphors, and their incomplete knowledge of natural phenomena. What was marvelous was thought miraculous. His 'forerunners,' his fastings, his diet, and manner of living, and that of his associates, all reveal the natural living, which brought him superior health with no need of any special divine assistance. He verified this by stating that future generations would 'do greater works than he did,' as they would get a better knowledge of natural—God's—'unchangeable' laws and methods. My 'coming book' will state, with convincing proof, that Christ's parentage, so-called miracles of healing, and apparent changes of natural law, his resurrection and ascension, into 'Heaven,' were in accord with natural law, but not then, and not wholly now, understood. The present ignorance of the laws underlying normal health is now, in this century, the greatest of all the past centuries, and is evidenced by the deterioration of the so-called civilized people, health-wise, although advanced far, in many ways. What I have learned by my researches and experiences, and the possibilities of restoring humanity to a superior health, with the advance of modern times, is like opening a 'Book of Seven Seals.' To show Christ's life in the sunlight of really natural and scientific laws, therefore eternal and really divine, identical with those of our own nature, is an inspiration and an aspiration which many are now enjoying and no one should miss.

"The other countries visited revealed phases and facts of natural health principles, and I took up with more confidence and enthusiasm than ever before the perfection of my own health by fasting experiments and an improved diet. I instinctively felt and

7

soon proved that certain natural foods prepared in the right way, had a superior energy producing power, and also a superior cleansing power, when rightly used, and in connection with an intelligent abstinence from any food, for the prevention as well as curing diseases of all kinds. That when used in accordance with the individual's encumbrance with disease debris—not germs—and their age, occupation, climate, season of the year, etc., that even the then so-called incurable diseases were helped in a uniform and orderly manner, and a cure certain, if not too much encumbered by habits and age. The *right* kinds and less food as a preparation for short or longer fasts as the condition indicated, gives the digestive organs a rest or "vacation" from over-work, and then the resuming of eating by a selection of the *right* kinds, (this being *very important*) brings wonderfully surprising and beneficial results. I fasted for twenty-four days with such marvelously pleasing results, not only to my physical condition, but to my mental and my aspirations spiritually, that my enthusiasm increased to tell my friends and other of my discoveries, experiences and conclusive results. I could not describe my feelings, but told them they must experience them for themselves, which some took up at once. I commenced my educational work by public fasts and lessons, fasting twice in large German cities, and twice in Switzerland. I was sealed in a room by Notaries of State, and strictly watched and controlled by physicians, and with no outside interference or communications. One fast of 21 days, one of 24, one of 32, one of 49 days in Cologne, all within a period of 14 months. Between these fasts, and after, my work was lecturing, giving tests of physical and mental efficiency, proving the value of what I had learned and experienced, and these forced me to teaching and advising others, writing articles, and starting a sanitarium in Switzerland, and advising by correspondence.

"My first written article was after my forty-nine day fast in Cologne, and published in a Vegetarian magazine, stating quite a new experience from fasting, diet and healing of disease; in fact, of life itself and in enjoyment and prolongation. It had a sensational and revolutionizing effect. It brought me letters of inquiry from all parts of the world, and in Europe particularly, health seekers, reformers and medical men were soon divided into opposers and enthusiastic followers. These writings brought on a scientific controversy or fight

8

over the new principles I had brought to light, that in Europe the two opposing combinations were known as 'Ehretists' and 'Non-Ehretists.'

"The *truth* of the Ehretists was well described by a prominent editor and reformer as follows: 'He (Ehret) did not invent or originate fasting, or the use of fruit or improved diet, for those are well known and were used long ago as good factors of Naturopathy, but what he did do was to originate an entirely new system of combining them as a systematic Healing method, on a basis of perfect Nutrition and Fasting.'

"My mucus theory—afterward a proven fact—as the fundamental cause of all diseases, was more and more recognized, and consequently my system of healing, too. It has stood the test and brought what one writer has expressed as 'enormous success,' and today has a platform that: *Natural Treatment and Diet is the Most Perfect and Successful* system of healing known. It has automatically named itself 'Nutro-Therapy' and its resulting movement 'Naturopathy.' For over ten years I wrote articles for health journals, lectured in the large cities of Europe, discussing the merits of the system with medical men and professionals, and treating thousands of patients at my 'Fruit and Fasting Sanitarium' and by correspondence, and without changing the fundamental principles, but strengthening them by a better knowledge of their details and how to apply them for best results. From all these was evolved what is now becoming well known in this country—the name, *'Mucusless Diet.'* I came to the United States just before World War I to visit the Panama Exposition, and to examine the fruits raised here, and particularly of California, and my enforced remaining here by the war has seemed providential in finding those here who had similar advances, discoveries and experiences, and we are now advocating and bringing to public knowledge the same principles that were so successful in Europe, in relieving suffering humanity and preventing disease, and developing an improved race of people that will not know what diseased conditions are, and bring about a better civilized humanity."

In editing Professor Ehret's life-work items, I am pleased to add that the discoveries made here by Dr. Thomas Powell, which I

9

assisted in developing and adding to, were intuitively surmised by Professor Ehret, and afterward found to be proved by his results, and later corroborated by reference to Chemist Hensel's scientific analysis of foods, are that fruits and vegetables have elements which are superior to those in any other foods, for producing vital energy, both in amount and quality. These elements or ingredients are known as "organized carbon" and "grape sugar." Their presence in sufficient quantities refutes the now current idea that the organic, mineral or tissue salts are the energy-producing elements. They exist only in infinitesimal amounts in all foods, and parts of them are drugs. Neither are the number of calories ("heat units" by calorimeter tests), reasonable basis for selecting a proper diet. My over forty years of observation, experiences and research have proven conclusively to me that fruits and vegetables have all the tissue salts needed, and that the presence of actually well-known ingredients in sufficient quantity are the energy and life supporting ingredients which make them the superior of all other foods, when the debris (mucus) from the "mucus-rich" foods is eliminated. Then the full beneficial effect of the "Mucusless Diet" can be enjoyed.

Prof. Arnold Ehret was undoubtedly one of the greatest healers of modern times—Philosopher, Teacher and Health Lecturer—he came to this country searching for further knowledge plus a desire to share his remarkable healing discoveries with those willing to accept.

This overwhelming desire to help his fellow humans—to learn the truth—together with a willingness to admit he did not know it all, was his motivating force. He recognized the necessity for united effort and hoped to avoid unpleasant consequences that result through petty jealousies. The valuable thoughts, deeds and words of wisdom were his heritage he left to us when he passed into the great beyond. The magnitude and versatility of the healing art that Prof. Ehret chose as his field of endeavor, welcomed the friendly cooperation of all Natural Healers and Drugless Practitioners.

More than any other thing, he wanted to give to the world the benefits of his now-proven health discoveries—this BETTER HEALTH which he himself had achieved and had already taught to thousands at this Swiss Sanitarium, public demonstrations, and through health magazine articles.

It was a constant source of personal gratification, to know that his health teachings were increasingly gaining acceptance among both the laity and professional practitioners as well—who unhesitatingly accepted fresh fruits and green leafy vegetables as the proper food for humankind. Even the personally coined descriptive words such as—"Mucus"—"Mucusless"—"Mucus-lean"—and "Mucus-plus" have gradually become well known.

Arnold Ehret leaves a heritage of vast worth to humanity—possibly the most important message that we have received since thousands of years! Ehret's teaching—vouchsafes to all his followers—HEALTH—which is more valuable than worldly wealth—joyous happiness in living—and a complete spiritual awakening! This humble message of mine, will hopefully bring added fame to a long-to-be-remembered "Apostle of Health"—Prof. Arnold Ehret.

–Prof. B.W. Child, c. 1924

Introductory

By Fred S. Hirsch

What is significant in all of Prof. Arnold Ehret's writings is that he had evidently a remarkable insight as to how man lived in the fabled paradisiacal Garden of Eden! It must at least be most certainly admitted that the man had visions which he found difficult to express into ordinary words. Surely, God's truth is as free as the water you drink, to all of us willing to partake of same at the fountain! And you will know exactly how to proceed, if only you have thoroughly acquainted yourself with the basic health teachings of Prof. Ehret.

First permit me to mention a few pertinent facts. Arnold Ehret was imbued solely with teaching his fellow man the proper methods of securing health, happiness and longevity through living in complete harmony with the laws of Nature! He achieved what others consider to be "seeming miracles"—and it now remains your privilege to judge for yourself whether the way of life taught by this long-to-be-remembered man with such deep convictions holds the promised health rewards for you! We have found it to be almost essential, as well as most desirable, to practically commit these teachings to memory:

1. Health is three-fold, i.e.: Body, Spirit and Soul!

2. Nature alone has the Power to Heal, and no other source possesses this Power!

13

3. When spiritually out of harmony, unhappily discontented, a complete change in mental attitude is necessary.

Revitalize through correcting the internal causes of ill health. Place your FAITH without reservations, in the power of Mother Nature to heal all ills, through proper diet. Know your body and spirit for they are the soul of humankind.

High ethical principles, spiritual aspirations, congenial work, fresh pure air, clean water and proper diet, forming the super-structure on which life is built.

Prof. Arnold Ehret has indicated the natural healing methods to be followed by those willing to join in raising a new civilization, where the individual will become more "precious" than the acquisition of "silver and gold." Feed your body "that which it needs" rather than that which it desires! The true attainment of life is mental and spiritual enfoldment, so "Let's Live Abundantly!" Following well-known, proven, natural laws will bring superior intelligence and superior health. We have become more ignorant of the Natural laws governing health in this supposedly enlightened century than we have ever been before in all of the past centuries. To live in accordance with the knowledge we presently possess; Natural laws, which are eternal, are an inspiration which certainly no one should miss. The Medical profession has tried in vain to suppress causes through treating the "symptoms" and we have blindly accepted the methods in general use today! Our body being the temple of the spirit—must be treated as an entity and not separately. Surgical removal of the offending organ, nor replacement of same through the process known as "transplantation" is not the answer! Only minor temporary relief, at best, can be achieved! The cleaner our temple is kept, the greater the spirit. REVITALIZE your body through correcting internal causes of illness.

Prof. Arnold Ehret has left to the world what might prove to be the most important message humankind has received during the past two thousand years! His health teachings vouchsafes for all of his followers, Health, Happiness in Living, and a complete Spiritual awakening!

—*Fred S. Hirsch, DNS. (Ehret Literature)*

14

Physical Fitness thru a Superior Diet, Fasting, and Dietetics

By Prof. Arnold Ehret

A strict interpretation of the word "Civilization" embraces spiritual culture, only, and its scientific meaning can be expressed as the ennobling and perfection of the human, in regard to his or her intellectual, moral and esthetic qualities.

In spite of this, we find that the highest degree of civilization in history (the classic period of the Hellenic Age) combined, or was even based upon a highly developed physical culture.

As a contrast, you may be reminded that the Middle Age is classified in the history of Christian civilization as a kind of spiritual stagnation—through its one-sided, nearly exclusive religious development, neglecting the culture of the body, entirely. Nietzsche may be somewhat right when he says, "Christianity has robbed us of the entire classic civilization." Saying this, he surely thought not only on the spiritual—but a great deal on the physical development of the classic Greek and Roman peoples.

The philosophy of Western Civilization is based upon Greek thinking, and the word treasure of all sciences has most of its roots in the Greek and Latin languages.

15

Esthetics, the science of beauty in the history of European art, especially sculpture and architecture, is based upon the Greek classic example of enduring foundation in principal lines.

There is no better example of the perfect human body than the Apollo and Venus of the classic Hellenic period, and the foot racers of the Marathon exemplify, undoubtedly, a classic example of physical culture.

The Greeks of this time were no doubt, cultivated and developed by physical training and a high standard of Eugenics.[1] The living models of the Gods were reproduced in sculpture by that great artist Phidias—the immortal creator of human beauty.

The gymnasium where unclothed boys and girls together received their daily physical exercise, as the principle of "classic education" is significant—as regards morals and education.

The "Temple of Aesculap," was mainly a place for what was known as "The Sleep in the Temple." Here all sick people would go, just as they go to a hospital today. They were kept "sleeping" all of the time—which properly translated means fasting.

Regarding the diet of the classic period, we know very little—but this much is certain, that is: Cooking and eating were not the most important things—as they are in this civilization. I do not suppose that at their banquets, which were called "Bacchanals," alcoholic beverages were used. In every artist's conception of this kind of a painting, the grapes are the "significant thing" at the "Bacchanal" festival.

I believe that a scholar of classic Greek language and civilization, of Greek philosophy, science, Greek art and mythology—one who

---

[1] Ehret used the term "eugenics" to make a philosophical point about the potential for developing an improved race of humans through the *Mucusless Diet Healing System*. For many modern readers, this term is off-putting due to its historical association with racist and genocidal policies in the United States, by Hitler in Germany, and throughout Western Europe. However, Ehret wrote this text before their infamous climax. Furthermore, Ehret's beliefs about a so-called superior race of people are diametrically opposed to the white supremacist mentality that was the foundation of most eugenic programs. (For more on this discussion, see notes from Lesson XXIV in the *Annotated, Revised, and Edited Mucusless Diet Healing System*.)

knows about and believes in physical culture—in fasting and dietetics—would at the same time find and discover this fact.

The classic age of Greek civilization—which we consider the highest in history—was due to and based upon a highly developed body through physical culture, fasting, dietetics and Eugenics. As with the Romans—degeneration set in just as soon as gluttony gained ground—as soon as Lucullus and Bacchus became Gods.

The production and development of individual bodily perfection and geniality was the goal of classic Greek civilization.

We find another standard of civilization existed with the ancient Egyptians, and it is said that their most prominent learned men and "High Priests" did not swallow solid foods for decades. They practiced "Fletcherism" some thousand years B. C.![2]

Seen through the glasses of dietetics and fasting—hygienic and dietetic rules—you will find that these same ideas run like a red string, through the Mosaic legislation, as well as through the stories of physical and spiritual heroes and prophets of the Old and New Testaments.

That physical culture in the classic age of ancient Greece was combined with fasting as well as a high standard of dietetics, can be proved by the stories of two of the greatest geniuses of history: Pythagoras and Hippocrates.

Pythagoras, an immortal mathematical genius, vegetarian and founder of a high-standing school of philosophy, went to Egypt to learn more about the "secret sciences" of that country. Before he was allowed to enter into the school of the learned, called High Priests at this time, he had to undergo a fast of forty days, under supervision, outside of the city. Believing that this was a test of his willpower and energy, he was told this: "Forty days' fast is necessary in order that you may grasp what we will teach you."

Hippocrates, another mathematician and learned in natural science, is today called the "Father of Medicine." He was the first to cleanse this "doctrine" from superstition and place it on a scientific

---

[2] "Fletcherism" is a method of eating developed by Horace Fletcher in which its practitioners are instructed to chew every bite of their food for 10 to 15 minutes.

basis. However, remarkable as it is—he practiced as an exclusive dietitian. He had very little knowledge of modern medicine, anatomy and physiology, yet he knew exactly what disease was, and what was taking place in the human body, during sickness. His ideas, concepts and teachings about how to heal every disease can be characteristically seen and understood by two quotations from his works on dietetics. He stated, "The more you feed the sick, the more you harm him." Also—"Your foods shall be your 'remedies,' and your 'remedies' shall be your foods."

His first statement proves clearly that he was an advocate of fasting and restrictive diet, especially in case of acute disease. His second statement (suggestion) embraces perfectly the entire problem of dietetics. It is exactly what I call the "Diet of Healing."

For a clearer understanding, it may be explained as follows: Nature's only and omnipotent "remedy"—fasting—is used in the animal kingdom to heal every disease and wound, showing that there is only one disease. I call it internal impurity—mucus derived from decomposed, un-natural foods. By healing wounds, Nature shows that she can do it better and more perfectly, without food.

In case of disease, Nature, with the instinctive "signal" of non-appetite, strives to say: "You did wrong by eating—stop it—or at least, replace the wrong foods which produced your disease, with good, clean, natural ones. You must do this, if I am to heal you and save you from the consequences of your wrong eating." Or, in the language of the Scriptures, "I am the Lord, thy Physician—my foods, produced by Nature only, are thy remedies—and thou shalt eat only the bread of Heaven—fruits and herbs [meaning green-leaf vegetables] (Genesis)."

For thousands of years—since the time of Hippocrates and Moses—the truth has been revealed, but not believed—not understood and not followed. Up to the present time, a "radical" diet, such as advocated by Hippocrates, as a diet of healing ("remedies")— and suggested by Moses, as humans' natural food, exclusively, has received little credit for healing ability—even among dietitians.

Why, in our time of regeneration by physical culture, have not fasting and dietetics become the principal and standard "remedy" of natural Therapeutics—as it was in the classic age of civilization, as shown above?

As a specialist in fasting and dietetics, with more than twenty years' practice, I submit this slow progress is due to the following facts: First, the modern person—the sick person, especially—is so overloaded with impurities, disease matters, that she cannot endure a long fast. In fact, it would, in many cases, become dangerous. My experience has taught me that shorter fasts, alternating with a cleansing diet, and progressively increased, are much easier and more successful than longer fastings. I call this process a systematical fast. Second: The radical fruit diet, the raw food diet, or, as I call it, the "Mucusless Diet"—(fruits, exclusively; nuts and green-leaf vegetables) stirs up and dissolves these poisons too rapidly in the body of the average sick person, with his lowered vitality—so much waste and toxemias that he cannot endure the elimination of the same. His condition becomes worse, instead of better, and he and everyone around him attribute it to the lack of solid food; and unfortunately for him his faith in natural foods has vanished, forever.

In fact, this is the reason why we have so much confusion in dietetics existing today. The amount of nutriment contained in a food is not the decisive point, but rather its eliminating qualities determine to what extent it is a "remedy"—according to Hippocrates.

I learned this, mostly, through my experience with serious cases of all kinds of disease and imperfect conditions. The change from wrong, disease-producing foods to right, disease-healing foods has to be effected slowly, progressively and systematically—according to the condition of the patient.

A diet of healing can never consist of recipes and the prescription of menus for the so-called different kinds of diseases. What I call the "Transition Diet" must be a therapeutic system of eating for elimination of waste and toxemias (disease matters) selected, adjusted and combined in such a way that the elimination can be controlled. Combined with fasting, we have a system of therapeutics that surpasses any other in existence.

If physical culture of any kind is combined with this system, the elimination can be enforced rapidly. After the body is once clean— free from any waste or poison—when all obstructions are removed from the human machine, then the physical culturist will develop a strength, endurance and a beauty of solid muscular proportion, and, at the same time, enjoy a mental and spiritual progress equaling that of the classic period of the "Hellenic Age."

No doubt our Western civilization is at stake. We drift along in a sort of semi-conscious condition—as though we were advanced to a high degree of civilization. The average mind thinks that the progress of technology and industry—economic and financial prosperity, and success, compose civilization. The flight (so-called escape) from healthful physical out-of-door work in the country, into the offices, theaters, restaurants, etc., located in the un-hygienic buildings of large cities, is considered progress.

Statistics show that we have the highest record in history in the development of consumption, cancer and syphilis. Whoever has treated chronic cases of this kind, knows the inside story of our so-called progress. Most of us believe we would benefit by getting from those that have more. How much more would it benefit us if we could only LEARN from those that KNOW more?

Due to the internal impurity of modern humans, their disease (of whatever nature) is of a degree never before attained by any people, in the history of humankind—and this is caused mainly, through their diet of civilization, and to the lack of physical culture.

At the present time we are menaced by an overwhelming culture of psychology; of metaphysics; of spiritualism—of spiritual "manias" of all kinds. It is significant that a well-known teacher of one of these cults had to remind his audience, upon different occasions, during the same lecture: "Yes; you must realize that you have a body." The spiritual confusion; the uncertainty and contradictions found even in science, philosophy and religion, have no analogy in the history of civilization.

The ignorance regarding the most important things in life—the health and perfection of the body—is indescribable. We suffer from a sort of psychic defect; failing to realize how important health is.

We are swimming in an ocean of books, and are brought into such a maelstrom of ideas that no one has a correct conception of the truth—or that health is the most important truth!

20

The attitude of the human mind toward everything spiritual is so terribly confused that you cannot find two people, today, who can agree on any one idea. This much is certain; however, there are no two truths about the spiritual and physical perfection of the human being. I have shown, through "classic examples," that the highest degree of real civilization—of mental and spiritual standards—was reached, and could be reached, only, through a most perfect body—through a superb, splendid health in every line—developed through physical culture, fasting, and dietetics.

The standard health of life is still based on the same facts that existed thousands of years ago—before humans learned how to start a fire—slaughter animals, and cook and bake them for food! Our food consisted solely of fruits and herbs, meaning green-leaf vegetables (see Genesis 1:29—the *Mucusless Diet*). You must believe these facts—and have unshakeable FAITH, in order to enable you to cure yourself! Secondly—you must learn that it will be necessary for you to go through a "cleansing" versus "healing" process, before you receive and can enjoy this paradisiacal nourishment. The only diet capable of producing an unknown high standard of health!

Cynics consider themselves realistic—but progress demands inspiration and motivation. If the individual will not banish all superstition from their mind, and properly take care of their body in every respect; they cannot be saved from disease and imperfection. What you get from life depends upon how much you want it.

Not many Western people realize the spiritual therapeutic value of fasting. But humankind, especially of the Western civilization, must soon take up the culture and care of the body, in the broadest sense—exactly as prevailed in the classic age of ancient Greece. The development of this process, physical fitness thru a superior diet,— will alone determine whether or not civilization can be saved!

- FINIS -

A Religious Concept of Physical, Spiritual, and Mental Dietetics

By Prof. Arnold Ehret

It had long been my desire to conduct a school dedicated to the teaching of the physiological transformation of humans; a new generation through the total elimination of every possible disposition for any 'disease' what-so-ever! A new type of human of Paradisiacal health, wisdom, beauty, happiness, of unchanging youth!

This was to be the key to the Paradise, the passage to a heaven on earth—this was to be a life of distinction—no more loss of hair, no decaying of teeth, wrinkle free, virile, mentally alert, no more presenility, a new, God-like human beyond the possibility of disease, and an aspiration for a longer-life with unlimited efficiency and endurance. Our goal may well encompass all of these muchly desired attainments!

The women of this new generation would be without menstruation, and pregnancy would be trouble free,—painless childbirth a matter of course and even predestination of the sex might be expected. Ample milk secretion a surety! Healthy disease-free babies without fear of children with intellectual disabilities, mental illness, or physical deformities! Imagine, if you will, a new type of children such as the growing of a new generation of physiological nobility of the blood, gaining prominence among their fellow humans through their physical appearance and by the grace of wisdom—

resulting through the cleanest of blood in hereditary selection. This was to be a school of divine healing with the message broadcast to all humankind throughout the world. Especially to those accepted leaders of today who, if they are to continue their present mode of life, can be expected to bring about the end of the society of humankind!

The Paradisiacal story has become almost completely misunderstood. The "apple" was never the forbidden food of humans, for the apple is in fact the ideal, the king of all fruits—the divine, the paradisiacal food. The real "bread of heaven." It was not the "apple," but the forbidden "false foods" representative of our present day adulterated, demineralized, commercialized synthetic foods—the accepted present day diet of civilization, that are the real physiological cause of all evils, symbolized by the sign of suffering—especially of the kinds of diseases produced by humans, that are driving them further and further away from a Paradisiacal existence.

A spiritual blindness has impelled our present "so-called" civilization to the current point of where it is rapidly becoming necessary to accept a sincere diet regime according to, and based on, our actual bodily requirements. It leads up to the solution of life's foremost problem, and it answers in the affirmative that great question; "Can we enjoy a paradisiacal existence on earth, or must all life be suffering?" We still have time to adjust to Nature's guidelines and re-establish our "Garden of Eden" so that humanity may once again live a natural, paradisiacal existence. To achieve this, humans must inevitably and intuitively return to the fruitarian diet, and through this change in both living conditions and food, will come a spiritual regeneration—a condition which can only be brought about after the "meek and humble" once again inherit the earth.

The cleansing must be two-fold—spirit and body. And only the inspired ones can appreciate and understand the fruitarian preference which is truly the divine paradisiacal food. The "chosen few" will listen and reap the rewards through the benefit of this knowledge and acceptance of these facts. Plainly stated, the facts can be listed as follows:

(1) Humanity's open rebellion against the laws of nature, as exemplified in our present age of living, cannot possibly endure!

(2) All is not lost as yet and we may firmly believe that it is possible that we may look forward to a rebirth of the "new-human" enjoying paradisiacal health with its unchanging youth! No more baldness or even graying of the hair. No more tooth decay and "false-teeth." Wrinkle free skin regardless of age. Unlimited endurance and total efficiency. The grace of wisdom and physical appearance assuring prominence among our fellow humans.

No one need expect to arrive at this condition of perfect health without first having gone through the "physiological fire of purification." A sort of "inner-burning" of the quantities of waste encumbrances contained in the body—acquired through years of wrong eating—especially the human-made, adulterated and chemically treated commercialized foods so prevalently in use today. Humankind has needlessly become sick and troubled because of these synthetic food-substitutes which are slowly but surely hastening the end of our Western civilization that cannot exist much longer in its present manner. We have in fact already entered the beginning of its dissolution.

The promised resurrection of humans as God-like beings can only be based on the divine laws of the reality of life and not on abstract ideas or an expectation of healing through miracles. A philosopher once said, "Education of man must begin 100 years before his birth." In the natural laws of producing ideal children— sons of God—not sickly and degenerate youth of today; the chosen ones will not be the sick in mind and body—they shall be those of Christ-like health. Intelligent, virile, handsome, affectionate—a new kind of race; not immoral degenerates planted in modern Sodoms, but in the garden of the new Eden!

We start the resurrection of humans by reconstructing the Paradise, planting fruit trees, vineyards and gardens—as our new residence. We bring not only a scientific system of healing based on Natural laws, but a regeneration,—a complete resurrection of the flesh,—by water, air—"spirit" (from the Greek word "Spiro" meaning air) and by the divine food of God—i.e. Fruits! It is the return of the oldest and yet the newest—of Adam the first man placed on earth—(as nearly as physiologically possible)—based on the laws of Nature, and acting today with the same absolute security as it did while Christ was first on earth some 2000 years ago, and as it undoubtedly did thousands of years before that! Fortunate is the person who has a strong abiding FAITH in which they can firmly believe! Every person must find their own, and the finding of it is important to each of us. Daily miracles are visible on every side; all evidence of the order and creation of which we are a part. FAITH helps us to mitigate fear and pain, to recognize and give thanks for our blessings. For after all—TIME is the great healer, and this is something on which we can positively count! The new 'God-like' men and women of Paradise can only be expected to return through physiological purification, and humankind's salvation requires healing from the "sins" of a civilization diet.

The mystery of Christ's coming on earth and His return to His Father, is a physiological problem of procreation. "Not only forth but up you shall plant yourself," said Nietzsche and I say, "The garden of love and matrimonium must be REAL fruit trees, nurtured under love ingredients, spreading flowers and perfumed roses." (High song of Solomon). The physiological problem of procreation and reproduction of higher, more perfect Adam-like beings—sons of God—is directed by God alone, the Father, the only One, original Producer of all humanity. The chosen ones will not be the "church runners"—those sick in mind and body, but they shall be of Christ-like health, a new kind of race; not planted in modern Sodoms, but in the garden of the new Eden. Only the true and faithful disciples of these teachings can qualify as the real and only ones in Christian history—of Christ's followers in fact!

We use the procreation of Christ from the physiological standpoint, as the divine law of purity in procreation—not conceived BY the Holy Spirit as a miraculous personality, but conceived IN the Holy Spirit—which means "in the sense of the Holy Spirit," the Natural laws of producing children—sons and daughters of God, and not sick and degenerated ones, like humankind of today.

Shall Christ really return to earth as a real, natural, reasonable fact—as a biological ideal of humans, as a true example of humankind's first man? That may and can happen only through Natural laws of procreation and laws of generation. He may come—

and by our reasoning, He can only again return not as His reincarnated soul of the same historical, identical personality,—but only in the sense of the return of the same!

The most tragic misunderstandings still cling over the centuries and the "Thirty Years' War" has His cause in the disputes, which arose over the question "Christ redeemed us by His blood." In the Lord's Supper He said, "This blood, which I drink is the blood of life for your salvation, through which you are resurrected," and "His blood" in the Lord's supper *was unfermented grape juice*. Physiologically the fruit of the grapevine is the nearest and best "blood food" of all healing, of "resurrection of life" at all. Through ignorance, or misunderstanding of these facts, as taught by science and all religions since the fall of Paradise—the life of humans has become a "tragedy of nutrition." The new God-like human can only result through physiological purification, through healing of humanity from the sins of the CIVILIZATION DIET, and the salvation and the Physiological Christianism which I firmly believe to be the true path to the paradise. This message is now deepened and glorified as an infallible truth through my conception of physiological religion.

THE CRITICAL POINT

From right or wrong eating, from much or less eating, depends on all beings. This fact is demonstrated in the animal kingdom. When an animal becomes sick or wounded, it instinctively uses the divine curative law of fasting, the contrary of eating. But, humans are the sickest beings on earth due to their loss of natural instinct, and the imaginary belief in a superior wisdom, and a resultant knowledge of food preparing.

Fasting is the most misunderstood and feared cure of all. Hundreds of self-styled fasting "experts" have published uncounted volumes about this subject, but nobody fully understands exactly what physiologically and pathologically happens when the "healing holy spirit," that is—the personal vital efficiency of the unfed body, purifyingly acts. Why is fasting so difficult, so weakening, and even so dangerous? Why is it so feared and so doubtfully undertaken? The answer is this mathematical, physiological formula: "V" equals "P" minus "O." Absolute Vital efficiency "V" is equal to air pressure "P" minus "O" obstruction (i.e.: mucus). Physically seen, the human body is an air-gas engine like that of every air machine which can operate a certain and relatively long time through air alone, which would mean in the case of a human being, absolute "activity" without food; i.e.: "air alone."[3]

The activity of every engine is equal to the impulsing power minus the resistance of friction. Air-power is activated everywhere exactly the same and therefore the vital efficiency of all humans should be the same throughout their life. Unfortunately this is not so, and this can only be caused by the difference of the resistance, of the obstruction of the latent foreign matters of disease. That is mucus, acquired through wrong diet, decayed, unused food stuffs. Mucus, proved and explained in my book *Rational Fasting for Physical, Mental, and Spiritual Rejuvenation*. Therefore, the more mucus in the system, the less the "vitality." Fasting means cleaning through the individual's own vitality. As soon as effects of the fast begin the bloodstream starts dissolving this mucus which is now deposited in the tissues of the entire system. Especially in the stomach and in the intestines, but expressly found in the organ suffering from the respective illness.

If there is a constitutional encumbrance of the entire system (full of mucus), the body cannot function since the obstruction is too great. No faster dies through lack of food, but rather through suffocation from his own "mucus," the real and final cause of death of all humanity. If the disease is at all curable, Nature heals not only the disease through a fast but it heals the whole person! Nature alone cures through that natural healing force which is self-curative, and which provides "Vitality" without food! The presence of foreign matter, waste encumbrances in the system, is "disease," gradually spreading over the entire body. Health is restored as soon as natural fruits and green-leaf vegetables replace the denatured foods.

---

[3] $V = P - O$ (Vitality equals Power minus Obstruction) is an equation devised by Arnold Ehret, which he calls the "formula of life." Ehret's proposition is that the human body is a perpetual-motion, air-gas engine powered exclusively by oxygen and that the body ceases to function when obstructed with waste. He asserts that mucus-forming foods create obstruction in the human body, and that a diet consisting of starchless/fat-free fruits and green, leafy vegetables are the only food that does not leave behind obstructive residues in the body and will aid it during the process of natural healing. For more, see "Lesson V" in *Prof. Arnold Ehret's Mucusless Diet Healing System: Annotated, Revised, and Edited by Prof. Spira.*

DISEASE AS AN EXPERIMENT

After curing myself from Bright's disease (after all other methods had failed), I commenced eating wrong foods again and my suffering soon came back. The same experience happened to several of my followers. Doubters can carry on similar experiments if they care to. No one need fear the recurrence of former ailments, just so long as they continue living on the proper corrective diet, and a rosy, youthful existence, free from all sickness, is assured them.

"Psychological Christianism" can be the most important event in the history of this Christian epoch. The errors of religion and so-called "science" are now discovered and must be overcome. For nearly twenty centuries Christianity has overlooked the care of the body and Christian humankind today suffers more than ever before. "Love thy neighbor" seems to have been completely overlooked and our record of self-destruction through warfare, murder and suicide, can be directly attributed to the present "civilization diet." Human's hoped for return to God's kingdom cannot and never will be realized through ethical and self-made morals, by praying and soft hearts, or by expecting "miracles," or through belief in transcendent existence. Christ was primarily a physician—not through the miracles he performed, but by natural laws of healing, and that is fasting and "divine foods," i.e. fruits! Through these teachings I bring you not only a system of healing constructed through scientific experiments and theories—but a message of regeneration. Resurrection of the flesh by water and air, (spirit—"spiro") and by the divine food of God, that is, fruit. All in accordance with and following the example of Christ, the greatest Master!

God's "heaven on earth" was originally in Paradise, the Garden of Eden, which literally means that human's living, eating, happiness, and absolute health has existed and can only again exist under "fruit-bearing trees" (See Genesis 1:29).[4] The promised resurrection as a God-like being is based on divine laws of reality of life and not on abstract ideas and miracles. But the key to Paradise is kept, and is symbolized by the fire sword of the angel. And as said by Christ, "Truly I tell ye, who is not regenerated by water and spirit will not come into the heaven." The true, real interpretation and physiologic truth of that pronouncement is, "Fasting." In other words, living by water and "spiro," i.e. air! Has not Christ given a record in fasting forty days in the desert?

I myself have fasted forty-nine days—a record in "watched and controlled" fasting. But to go still further, nobody arrives at an exclusive, satisfying, perfectly nourishing, fruit diet without having first prepared themselves through a long fast, and gone through the "physiological fire of the purification," the "burning" of the morbid matters in his body acquired from "sins" of wrong eating. The fall of humanity is a "sin of Diet."

The resurrection of humanity through Christ's teachings and in accordance with His own example of the "re-newed" Adam together with a resurrection of the lost paradise as our residence, has already started! Added proof that we, and we alone, are the only real followers of His teachings.

When humans were originally placed by their Maker in a paradisiacal garden with its abundance of fruit trees and green leaf herbs, God provided also invisible food—consisting of pure, undefiled fresh air (the breath of life), laden with the aroma from flowering shrubbery and luxuriant foliage of plants and trees. Clear, sparkling water, running streams, unpolluted by human-made poisonous chemicals, were available year round for humans to quench their thirst—and the magnetic impulses together with electrical vibrations coming direct from the solar rays furnished vital

---

[4] **Genesis 1:29 (Bible)**: The voice of God tells Adam and Eve that their diet should consist of fruit: "And God said, Behold, I have given you every herb [plant] bearing seed, which is upon the face of all the earth, and every tree, in which is the fruit of a tree yielding seed: to you it shall be for food [meat]." (Vulgate translation). According to this verse, the fruit of a tree yielding seed, as well as the seeded fruit from herbs (plants such as a grapevine), are to be the food of humans. For more, see the note section of "Lesson I" in the *Prof. Arnold Ehret's Mucusless Diet Healing System: Annotated, Revised, and Edited by Prof. Spira.*

forces for the body. And the good earth added its share of these "invisible foods" for both spirit and body, which are inexorably interconnected and require these essentially necessary vital forces for life.

We continually seek physiological regeneration and eventually find that the key to paradise and its paradisiacal health is fundamentally obtainable only through a complete redemption (salvation) from all evils. A physiological regeneration by the "bread of heaven," i.e. fruits and starchless green-leaf vegetables. And even this "heavenly food" must first pass through the purgatory of the stomach and intestines before being accepted!

Since the fall of the Paradise, science as well as all religions, with the possible exception of a very few, have as yet failed to arrive at a complete understanding of this basic truth: "Humankind has become a victim of the tragedy of nutrition." Or could it be through total ignorance?

The new God-like human that we envision possessing an unlimited amount of vital force, will be beyond the possibility of sickness or disease of any kind. Residing in their reconstructed paradise, the abode of the intelligent "chosen-ones," and existing solely in accordance with the biological law of eating as taught in Genesis 1:29 (fruit alone, the infallible food of humans).

A religious group which existed during the time of Christ was known as the "Essenes" and the members practiced asceticism, particularly in diet. They were principally fruitarians and were viewed as "holy men" because of their wisdom. During their infrequent visits to the villages they were accepted in a most cordial manner and were highly respected by everyone in the community through recognition of their scholarly achievements. Consulted and sought after for guidance and advice on all important matters, their friendship was highly prized by all. It is said that Christ, during His youth, was tutored and received His education from them, which undoubtedly accounts for His thorough knowledge of the holy scriptures exemplified in all of His messages which have now spread all over the entire world! Christ was primarily a physician—not because of the miracles which He performed on the sick; but through His

31

teachings of the natural laws of healing: i.e., fasting and diet—the divine foods—fruits and the natural green leaf starch-less vegetables.

My *Mucusless Diet Healing System* is therefore a return of the oldest and yet the "newest!" It is a return to the first man, or as nearly as is physiologically possible today, all in accordance with and closely following the examples of Christ Himself. The teachings of the *Mucusless Diet Healing System* are constructed and based upon scientifically proven and recognized theories. A complete resurrection and regeneration of the flesh through water and air (spiro/spirit), together with the divine God-given foods. If proof is needed that the teachings of the Mucusless Diet are closely aligned with the teachings of Christ, based on the laws of nature, surely this is a most convincing proof! For it acts today with the same absolute security—just as it functioned 2000 years ago! Furthermore, Christ, whether He has existed or not, is the highest, the most divine example of man ever produced. Not only was Christ the son of God, but the most perfect of all God's sons. If we are to recognize this revelation as did the prophets of old, then we too must undergo a purifying of the brain-cells, which can only be accomplished through fasting.

Drugless practitioners have achieved over the centuries almost miraculous results in healing the sick, using only natural methods in various ways. Toleration for their beliefs and teachings have always been received with an open mind, and their achievements duly noted—but acceptance came slowly. The valuable thoughts, deeds and words of wisdom, left by those who have long ago passed into the great beyond, bring us conclusive proof of the versatility and magnitude of Natural healing. Many of our leading scientists, including those of the highest scholastic accomplishments, as well as practically all of the medical practitioners of today, appear unimpressed by Nature's healing abilities—preferring to place their faith in medical drug concoctions and the surgeon's scalpel through removal of the "offending organ." Disease, sickness and suffering, in fact all of the ailments presently known to humanity can be eliminated and completely overcome through the biological law of eating fruit alone, the infallible, true food for humans! It has now been long realized and recognized that abstention from food of any kind brings humans closer to the spiritual realm—advances their well-being through increased vitality with the resultant prolongation of life itself.

And here are a few secrets I learned through my own fasting experience: After a preparative diet you fast easily with more enjoyment in both bodily and mental experience. Only after this longer fast (i.e., two or three weeks) is the taste completely acquired for an exclusive fruit diet, satisfying and perfectly nourishing. Then, through this experience only, will you become convinced that fruit is the most perfect of all foods. Most persons and even many doctors believe, because of their complete ignorance of what physiologically takes place when a 'meat-eater' eats one or two fruit meals, that serious results can happen.

We need a purifying of the brain—through fasting—to recognize as did the prophets of old "the revelation." You cannot pass the gate watched over by the angel with the flaming sword until you have gone through the purgatory (cleansing fire) of fasting and a diet of healing. A cleansing—a physiological purifying by the "Flame of Life" in your own body! During thousands of years, no one has escaped the struggle of death caused by an unnatural life, and you will eventually have to face it someday. All disease of humankind, both mental and physical, ever since the dawn of civilization have the same foundational cause—regardless of what the symptoms may be. It is without exception, one and the same general condition—a oneness of all disease, namely waste, foreign matter, filth, mucus and its poisons.

The vital efficiency of all humans should remain the same during their entire life, and as a follower of the Ehret health teachings you will have learned that every mouthful of wrong food eaten becomes an obstruction in the bodily machine—an encumbrance, a restriction of your vitality, strength and endurance. Regardless of how small it may seem at the time, it is an interference with your standard of health. Disease of every kind is no longer a mystery for you, and so it may come as a "shock" when I state the tragic fact that almost all individuals living today—and this includes the most learned and highly educated college professors, scientists, doctors and lawyers, artists, politicians and business leaders, and many others—live in darkest ignorance about the most important thing in life—i.e., their health! It is bordering on the ridiculous and yet tragic, that our source of information on this important subject should be furnished by the medical fraternity who actually teach through ignorance—"How to eat your way to illness!" Medications and drugs of all kinds may well be used to suppress pain and symptoms of disease, but suppression can only lead to more serious physical instability with possible fatal results. Natural treatments—so-called because no drugs are used—are indeed more or less cleansing as well as healing. But, natural treatments fail to stop the source of supply, that is the "diet of civilization" which is the fundamental cause of most illness, whatever be its name. All of the animal kingdom suffer through "over-eating" at times. This fact is demonstrated by domesticated animals as well as those living in their wild state. If any animal is sick or wounded, it instinctively follows the divine, curative law of fasting, the contrary of the evil-causing overeating. And the fasting continues until health returns. But humans who consider themselves to be smarter than all others, with their skilled knowledge of food preparation, are the sickest beings of all, and fasting is misunderstood and feared. When the healing "holy spirit"—that is to say—the personal vital efficiency of the unfed body purifyingly acts, no one seems to understand what is physiologically and pathologically actually taking place.

But you, I and all others who have learned this greatest and most important truth of life and have embraced these teachings, in fact and not by mind only, are out of the "road of darkness," and into the light of the new civilization—a superior physical regeneration, the foundation of mental and spiritual progress.

This is an outline of the serious nature of this work, upon which depends not only your future destiny, but that of a suffering, unhappy humankind, teetering on the verge of a physical and mental collapse.

- FINIS -

34

The Enforcement of Elimination by Physical Adjustments: Exercises, Sunbaths, Internal Baths, and Bathing

From Lesson XXV, An Excerpt from Prof. Arnold Ehret's Mucusless Diet Healing System: Annotated, Revised, and Edited by Prof. Spira

As shown in previous lessons, all physical treatments vibrate or shake the tissues and thereby stimulate the circulation in one way or another for the purpose and with the result of loosening and eliminating "foreign matters," the cause of all diseases.[1] The human body does this itself, in the most perfect way, as soon as you fast or as soon as your blood composition has been changed by natural diet.

Physical treatments and physical culture can therefore be combined with this diet and fasting to enforce and to hasten the elimination. However, I must advise that extreme care be taken not to exaggerate, especially on "bad" days—days of strong elimination. If you are tired and you feel bad, then rest and sleep just as much as you can. On the days that you feel "good" during a fast or strict diet, you may take some physical treatment also, such as exercise, baths, massage, deep breathing, etc.

The most natural exercises, and by far the best, are walking, dancing, and singing. The latter is the most natural breathing exercise with the added advantage of loosening chest vibrations.[2] An excellent "exercise," and one that everybody knows, is hiking in the mountains.

When climbing hills, you increase your breathing in the most natural way. Your breathing becomes better and more harmoniously than with any "system" of exercises.

The cleaner you become the more easily you will understand what I teach in Lesson V—that air and the other ingredients of the forests are "food"—invisible food.

Both hands should be free when walking, so as to permit continually the natural movements.

Outdoor garden work is another natural exercise.

By taking proper care of your body, you will generate health. The following exercises are suggested for those who desire to keep physically fit. I must again remind you that air is more necessary to life than food. Proper breathing is therefore essential. *Do not exercise in a close, stuffy room.* Stand before an open window. Take a deep, full breath with each exercise. Inhale through nose and expel through mouth. Stand before a mirror while exercising, and admire the suppleness and graceful manner in which you perform each movement. Fall in love with yourself if no one else will. Keep the feet about 15 inches apart—stand erect and use muscular tension.

Exercise No. 1

Standing erect, hands to the side, clench the fists tightly. Raise arms slowly as high above the head as possible, taking a deep breath. Relax and expel breath. Repeat five times.

Exercise No. 2

Extend arms and ensure that your arms are at your chest level. Grasp hands tightly and pull to the right side, resisting with left hand. Then go through the same motion pulling to the left side. Relax after each motion, expelling breath. Repeat each exercise five times.

Exercise No. 3

Grasp the left hand firmly with the right, in front of body. Resisting with the left hand, lift with the right, using full strength while raising the arms high above your head. Take deep breath on the upward motion, and relax before expelling. Repeat with the right hand resisting with the left, five times each.

Exercise No. 4

Clasp hands above the head, allowing them to rest on your head. Bend to the right side, pulling hard, then to the left five times, and then alternate first right and then left. Between each movement take a deep breath and expel when relaxed. This exercise is especially good for stimulating the liver.

Exercise No. 5

Clasp hands in back of neck, holding all muscles tense. Twist to the right, then to the left five times. Now pull to the right and then to the left five times. Now pull to the left and then to the right five times. Hold your legs rigid, but permit your body to sway.

Exercise No. 6

Grasp the hands behind the back and without bending the body, raise arms up as far as possible. Inhale on the upward motion; relax and expel. Repeat five times. This exercise is for developing the chest.

Exercise No. 7

Place your right hand over your right hip, clench left fist, and raise left arm slowly, taking a deep breath. At the same time, bend the body as far to the right as possible. Make it hurt. Relax and expel breath. Repeat with left hand placed on hip, and raising right arm with fist tightly clenched. Repeat each five times.

Exercise No. 8

Grasp hands firmly in front of breast, all muscles tense; and twist to the left. Now twist to the right as far as possible. Do not permit feet to move. Inhale during motion; relax and expel breath. Repeat each exercise five times.

Exercise No. 9

Raise arms above the head as high as possible, even permitting body to bend backward. Now bend body forward and without bending the knees try to touch the floor with your fingers. Exhale breath when relaxed. Repeat this exercise slowly five times, and gradually increase to 20 times.

Do not exhaust yourself in any of the exercises. If the exercises make you stiff at first, it is a sure sign that you needed them, and that they are doing you good. The soreness will soon wear off if you continue the exercises persistently. You may add other exercises to these, but be sure they have the deep breathing. *Play your favorite music when exercising.* Any snappy march piece will do.[3] The vibrations from the music are wonderful. It is preferable to exercise the first thing in the morning—immediately upon arising. If clothing is worn, it should be loose. Start with a few exercises at first and then increase gradually. Above all things, do not consider it a duty, but put fun into them. Dancing alone and bending movements to the accompaniment of music will prove very beneficial.

Sunbaths

Whenever you have an opportunity of doing so, take a sunbath. In the beginning, do not exceed 20 to 30 minutes and keep the head covered. On "bad" days—days of great elimination—stay cool.

The cleaner you become, the more you will enjoy the sunbath and the longer you will remain. You will also find that you can stand it much warmer. A short cool shower or a cool rub with a towel dampened in cold water immediately after the sunbath is good.

The sunbath is an excellent "invisible" waste eliminator, and it rejuvenates the skin, causing it to become silk-like and coloring it a natural brown. Civilized humans of our race show by their white skin that they are sick from birth on; they inherit the mucused, white blood corpuscles—the "sign of death."

As all of the clothing should be removed during a sunbath, a small enclosure just long enough to lie in should be built in your backyard, or even on the roof, away from prying, inquisitive eyes. The clothing of civilization has made it impossible for humans to secure their proper quota of the life-giving power of fresh air and sunshine, so essential to health and happiness. The direct rays of the sun on the naked body supply the electricity, energy, and vitality to the human storage battery, renewing it in vigor, strength, and virility.[4]

Internal Baths

During the transition period, even though you have regular bowel movements, *it is advisable to wash out the lower colon.* The sticky waste,

40

slimy mucus, and various poisons which Nature is attempting to eject should be helped along as much as possible. A small-bulb infant syringe can be used after the regular bowel movement, but for a thorough cleansing, two to three quarts of water should be used.[5]

Try to have a natural bowel movement before injecting the water. The body should be in a reclining position, lying on the right side.[6] The syringe must not be higher than three or four feet above the patient. Water should be warm, not hot, and it should be tested on your elbow. Should any discomfort be felt, stop the flow until the discomfort passes as the entire two or three quarts should be retained at one time. If the cramp or pain becomes too great, allow the water to pass from the colon and repeat the operation.

The water should remain in the intestines for about 15 or 20 minutes, or as long as it is comfortable. While still lying on your side, gently massage the colon in an upward motion. Then lie on the back with the knees drawn up and massage from right side of body to left; now turn over, lying on the left side, and massage the left side with a downward motion. You should now be ready for ejecting the water. The best time to take an enema is just before retiring.

Bathing

Authorities differ on bathing almost as widely as they do on diet. The *Mucusless Diet Healing System* will produce the "skin you love to touch" through clean blood supply, and without the aid of cosmetics, lotions, and cold creams.

It is not necessary to take a daily hot bath with soap and brush under ordinary conditions.

The morning "cold shower" during the entire year, without any consideration of weather conditions, is also inadvisable. There is no need to deliberately subject the body to an extreme shock, and in a number of cases more harm than good may result.

Needless to state, the skin must be kept clean so that the pores may be permitted to properly function, and this can be accomplished by the following method:

Place a basin of cool water before you. Dip the hands in the basin and starting with the face, rub briskly; wet the hands again and apply to the neck and shoulders; next rub the chest and stomach; next the arms and then the back, and last the legs and feet. Put the feet right into the basin if you care to. Keep moistening the hands as needed, but there is no necessity for throwing any quantity of water on the body. To dry off, rub with the bare hands for 5 minutes if possible, until the body is all aglow, or wipe with a towel. This should be done upon arising immediately after you have taken your exercises. The results will surprise you. If you prefer a tub bath, then allow about one inch of cold water to run into the tub. Sit in it with knees drawn up, and follow the same rule of rubbing and massage as outlined above.

Remember that the air bath is just as essential as the water bath. A few minutes each day spent before an open window, upon arising and just before retiring, when all clothes are removed, massaging the body—help the skin to retain its natural functioning qualities.[7]

Always bear in mind that extremes of any kind are harmful. This applies to exercise, bathing, and sleeping, as well as extremes in eating. Even extreme joy and happiness has been known to kill just as readily as extreme anger, hate, and worry. Therefore, AVOID EXTREMES OF ALL KINDS.

Notes by Prof. Spira:

[1] Ehret does not advocate excessive exercise for the purposes of loosening and eliminating waste. Historically, there have been various therapies that use intensive shaking and massage as a primary means to loosen waste. For Ehret, rational and natural physical activity is best, and excessive exercise and massage should be avoided.

[2] Practicing the "Science of Breath" or rational forms of yoga go hand-in-hand with the mucusless diet.

[3] Feel free to listen to something other than marches if you are moved to do so. Historically, marches became one of the most popular forms of music around the world throughout the 1800s and early 1900s. Before the advent of phonograph records, if people wanted to hear music they had to either make it themselves or see it performed live. The military band craze of the 1800s is even partly responsible for the marching bands that still play a visible role in school and university music programs. With that said, Ehret was a man of his times, and the prospect of exercising to a phonograph record was innovative and exciting.

⁴ The power of sunbathing to aid the body in cleansing must not be underestimated. It is recommended to not use sun-blocking lotions, which terribly constipate the pores. As with all aspects of the diet, be sure to transition into longer periods in the sun. The cleaner you become, the easier it will be to safely and naturally lavish in the hot sun for long periods of time.

⁵ Two or three quarts of water is the amount that fits in most standard enema bags. Many modern-day mucusless diet practitioners use lemon juice and distilled water enemas regularly or as needed. For more details about doing enemas, see the section on lemon juice enemas in *Spira Speaks: Dialogs and Essays on the Mucusless Diet Healing System*.

⁶There are different schools of thought about what is best to lie on. For a more detailed discussion, see the lemon enema section in *Spira Speaks: Dialogs and Essays on the Mucusless Diet Healing System*.

⁷ A good rule of thumb is to not put anything on your skin that you would not be prepared to eat. Soap, makeup, lotions, deodorant, etc., all enter your body through your pores. It is recommended to find soaps etc. made with the most natural ingredients. Many supermarkets now carry natural hygiene products in their "organic" or "natural" foods sections. It is strongly recommended that you avoid using standard deodorants, which terribly clog up the pores of your underarms. Armpit odor comes from one of two sources: 1) the stench of internal wastes or 2) bacteria tucked away in the outside of your pits. The former source radically decreases as you cleanse your insides of putrid waste. For the latter, I have found **lemon juice underarm air baths** to be the greatest way to safely eliminate foul odor from the outside of the body. Juice one lemon, then take a clean cloth or paper towel (all natural with no inks is preferable) and sop up some of the juice. Then apply it to your underarms, one at a time. Afterword, raise your arms toward the sky for several minutes and let the lemon juice air-dry. Letting the oxygen dry the juice helps to eliminate all odor-causing agents. This method can be much cheaper and less harmful than using store-bought deodorants or antiperspirants.

(Many mucusless diet practitioners buy lemons, and other items, in bulk from local grocers or fruit and vegetable wholesalers. Wholesalers often have "cash-and-carry" options and will be willing to sell you boxes of fruits and vegetables for the whole family.)

A Message to Ehretists

Dear Friends:

After careful and intelligent study of the foregoing lessons, you now know that disease consists of an unknown, decayed, and fermented mass of matter in the human body, decades old—especially in the intestines and colon. You likewise know how unwise and ignorant it is to think that knowing what to eat is, alone, a complete diet of healing.

None of the recognized authorities know the tremendous importance of a thorough and deep cleansing of the human "cesspool." All are more or less "fooled" by nature when they advise eating of fruits, with stomach and intestines clogged up by mucus and decomposed protein foods, eaten from childhood onward right into adulthood and beyond.

You have been taught the result: should these poisons—cyanide of potassium—be dissolved too rapidly and be permitted to enter the circulation, severe sensations—even death—may occur, and humanity's natural food, oranges, grapes, dates, etc., are blamed!

My teachings clearly prove that this hitherto unexplained ignorance regarding fruit diet is the "stumbling-block" for all other food research experts, who have made personal experimental tests. I have heard the same cry thousands of times and even from young and supposedly healthy persons—"I became weak!" And all experts,

45

with the exception of I, say, "Yes, you require more protein; at least eat nuts."

During my personal tests involving this same problem, I tried to overcome this "stumbling-block" hundreds of times. After a 2-year cure in Italy of Bright's disease with consumptive tendency, by fasting and strict living on a mucusless diet, I ate two pounds of the sweetest grapes and drank half a gallon of fresh, sweet grape juice, made from the best and most wonderful grapes grown there. Almost immediately, I felt as though I were going to die! A terrible sensation overcame me, palpitation of the heart, extreme dizziness which forced me to lie down, and I was seized with severe pains in the stomach and intestines. After 10 minutes, the great event occurred— a mucus-foaming diarrhea and vomiting of grape juice mixed with acid-smelling mucus, and then the greatest event of all! I felt so wonderfully well and strong that I at once performed the knee-bending and arm-stretching exercises 326 times consecutively. All obstructions had been removed!

For the first time in history, I have shown what humans were when they lived without "fired" foods—during the prehistoric times (called Paradise) eating fruits, the "bread of heaven."

For the first time in human history, this "demon" in the tragedy of human life has been shown—and how they can and must be eliminated—before men and women can again ascend to a Paradisiacal health, happiness, immunity from disease and "God-like" being.

If the Garden of Eden—heaven on earth—ever existed it must have been a "fruit orchard." For thousands of years, through wrong civilization, humans have been tricked into unconscious suicide, reduced to slavery, to produce wrong food, "earning their bread by the sweat of their brow." Unnatural foods cause sickness and death.

"Peace on Earth" happiness and righteousness as yet remain a foolish dream. During thousands of years, God, Paradise, Heaven— Sin, Devil, Hell—seldom found an interpretation that a clear, reasoning mind would willingly accept. The average unfortunate fellowman thinks of God as a good and forgiving Father who will allow him to enter Paradise in another world—unpunished for any violations of His laws in nature.

46

I have proven for the first time in history that the diet of Paradise is not only possible—good enough for degenerate humankind, such as we now are—but that it is the Unconditional Necessity and the first step to real salvation and redemption from the misery of life. That it is a needed key to the lost paradise where disease, worry, and sorrow—hate, fight, and murder—were unknown, and where there was no death, from unnatural causes at least.

"We are what we eat" is a philosopher's greatest and truest statement.

You must now see why civilization, all religion, all philosophy, with their tremendous sacrifice of work, time, money, energy, are and have been part guesswork. The magic formula for "Heaven on Earth"—of the Paradise—must read like this:

"Eat your way into Paradise physically." But you cannot pass the gate, watched over by the angel with the flaming sword, until you have gone through purgatory (cleansing fire) of fasting and diet of healing—a cleansing, a physiological purifying, by the "Flame of Life" in your own body! For thousands of years no one has escaped the struggle of death caused by an unnatural life, and you will have to face it someday.

But you, I, and others who have learned this greatest and most important truth of life, are the only ones in existence today who are in fact, and not by mind only, out of the road of darkness and unconscious suicide and into the light of the new civilization—the light of a physical regeneration—as the foundation of mental and spiritual revelation-like progress to the light of a superior, that is to say, a spiritual world.

This book represents an outline of the serious nature of my work and it also appeals to you for help in carrying it through as the greatest deed you can perform—upon which depends not only your future destiny, but that of a suffering, unhappy humankind—on the verge of physical and mental collapse.

ARNOLD EHRET

About Prof. Spira

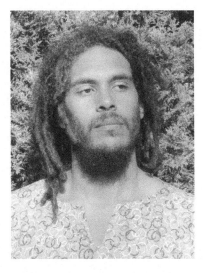

In 2002, Prof. Spira was a 280-pound former varsity high school football player suffering from multiple ailments such as daily migraine headaches, allergies, regular bouts of bronchitis, sleep apnea, persistent heartburn, etc. After having lost his mother to a terrible string of chronic illnesses when he was in the 6th grade, he grew up assuming that he was genetically destined to be sick his whole life. While studying jazz trombone performance at the University of Cincinnati's College Conservatory of Music, he met a jazz drummer named Willie Smart (aka Brother Air) who told him about Arnold Ehret's *Mucusless Diet Healing System*. Within 6 months of reading the book, Spira lost 110 pounds and overcame all of his major ailments. He was able to throw away his CPAP unit (an oxygen mask that treats sleep apnea) and the medications he had taken since childhood. Since his transformation, he has worked tirelessly to revive Arnold Ehret's teachings and has helped thousands of people learn how to transition toward a mucus-free lifestyle.

Spira is a professional jazz trombonist, educator, and author. He holds a Master of Music in jazz trombone performance from the University of Cincinnati's College-Conservatory of Music, a Master of Arts in African American and African Studies, and a Doctor of Philosophy in musicology with a specialization in ethnomusicology from the Ohio State University. He is also the co-leader of an all-vegetarian and Ehretist jazz group entitled the Breathairean Ensemble, whose members are dedicated to inspiring their listeners to pursue what they call "physiological liberation."

In 2014, Spira created Mucus-free Life LLC, which currently publishes several books including Prof. Arnold Ehret's *Mucusless Diet Healing System: Annotated, Revised, and Edited by Prof. Spira*, *Spira Speaks: Dialogs and Essays on the Mucusless Diet*, *Prof. Arnold Ehret's Rational Fasting*, *Definite Cure of Constipation*, and *Thus Speaketh the Stomach*. In Spring 2016 he released the first audiobook format of his acclaimed annotated version of *Arnold Ehret's Mucusless Diet* and plans to release a revolutionary *Mucusless Diet eCourse* this year. He is the webmaster of www.mucusfreelife.com, facilitates popular public support groups for Mucusless Diet practitioners, and produces educational videos about the *Mucusless Diet* on his YouTube Channel.

List of Other Publications

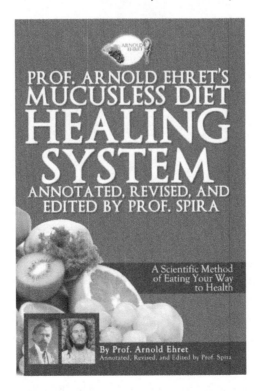

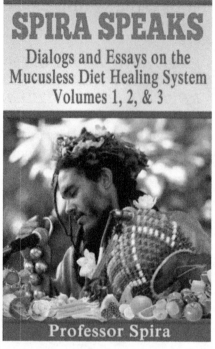

Join Prof. Spira for an unprecedented look into the healing power of a mucus-free lifestyle! After losing 110 pounds and overcoming numerous physical ailments, Spira learned that he had a gift for articulating the principles of the diet through writing and music. As he began to interact with health-seekers on the internet in 2005, he realized that written dialogs about the diet could benefit far more than just their intended readers. This book is a compilation of the best writings by Professor Spira on the subject.

What is the *Mucusless Diet Healing System*? How has it helped numerous people overcome illnesses thought to be permanent? What does it take to practice a mucus-free lifestyle in the twenty-first century? Why is the transition diet one of the most misunderstood aspects of the mucusless diet? Spira answers these questions and much more in his unprecedented new book that contains never-before released writings about the mucusless diet.

Visit www.mucusfreelife.com/spira-speaks

Prof. Arnold Ehret's Rational Fasting for Physical, Mental, and Spiritual Rejuvenation: Introduced and Edited by Prof. Spira

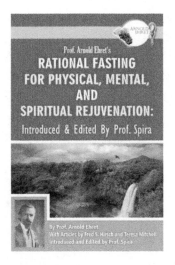

Discover one of Ehret's most vital and influential works, the companion of the Mucusless Diet Healing System. Introducing *Rational Fasting for Physical, Mental, and Spiritual Rejuvenation: Introduced and Edited by Prof. Spira*, now available from Breathair Publishing.

In this masterpiece, Ehret explains how to successfully, safely, and rationally conduct a fast in order to eliminate harmful waste from the body and promote internal healing. Also included are famous essays on Ehret's teachings by Fred Hirsch and long-time devotee Teresa Mitchell.

You will learn:

- The Common Fundamental Cause in the Nature of Diseases
- Complete Instructions for Fasting
- Building a Perfect Body through Fasting
- Important Rules for the Faster
- How Long to Fast
- Why to Fast
- When and How to Fast
- How Teresa Mitchell Transformed Her Life through Fasting
- And Much More!

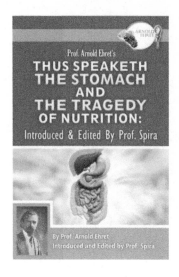 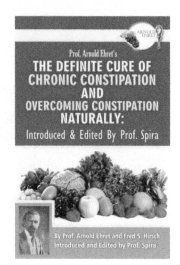

Thus Speaketh the Stomach and The Tragedy of Nutrition

If your intestines could talk, what would they say? What if you could understand health through the perspective of your stomach? In this unprecedented work, Arnold Ehret gives voice to the stomach and reveals the foundation of human illness.

The Definite Cure of Chronic Constipation and Overcoming Constipation Naturally: Introduction by Prof. Spira

In *The Definite Cure of Chronic Constipation and Overcoming Constipation Naturally*, Prof. Arnold Ehret and his number-one student Fred Hirsch explore the generally constipated condition of the human organism.

COMING SOON!!!

The Art of Transition: Spira's Mucusless Diet Healing System Menu and Recipe Guide

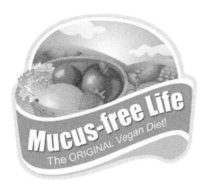

What does a mucusless diet practitioner actually eat? What kind of transitional mucus-forming foods are best? What are the most effective menu combinations to achieve long-lasting success with the mucusless diet? What are the best transitional cooked and raw menus? What foods and combinations should be avoided at all costs? How can you prepare satisfying mucusless and mucus-lean meals for your family?

These questions and much more will be addressed in Prof. Spira's long-awaited mucusless diet menu and recipe eBook! Stay tuned!

Introduction

Purpose

Popular Fruits, Vegetables, and Vegan Items Omitted from this Book

Organic vs. Non-Organic

Mucus-Lean

Raw vs. Cooked

Satisfying Nut and Dried Fruit Combinations

The Onion Sauté

Filling Steamed and Baked Vegetable Meals

Spira's Special "Meat-Away" Meal

Mucusless

Raw Combination Salads

Raw Dressings

Favorite Mono-Fruit Meals

Favorite Dried Fruits

Favorite Fruit Combinations

Vegetable Juices

Fruit Smoothies and Sauces

Fresh Fruit Juices

Sample Combinations and Weekly Menus

Projected Release: Spring 2019

SPIRA'S MUCUSLESS DIET

COACHING & CONSULTATIONS

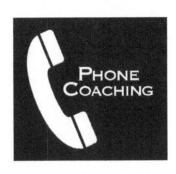

"After receiving a consultation with Professor Spira, I was able to take my practice of the Mucusless Diet Healing System to a new level. Speaking face to face with an advanced practitioner was key and a true blessing on my journey. I'm looking forward to following up with another in the future!"

—*Brian Stern, Certified Bikram Yoga Instructor and Musician*

"You truly are amazing. You have done nothing but given all you can to help me and I truly appreciate this. Thank you for 'feeding me.'"

—*Samantha Claire, Pianist and Educator*

"Spira has experienced cleansing on a higher level and passes those experiences to us. He teaches us by EXAMPLE and not only by WORDS, which is rare to find in the world we live in."

—*Georgia Barretto, Brazilian Jazz Musician*

"When I came across Prof. Arnold Ehret's Mucusless Diet Healing System: Annotated, Revised, and by Prof. Spira *it was an epiphany because I finally understood the root cause of human illness, and therefore the compensation action that must be taken to correct prior years of wrong disease-producing foods that have been eaten since birth."*
—*Andrae K. Genus, M.Sc., Environmental Scientist and Holistic Health Expert*

Spira has practiced the mucusless diet and studied the natural hygienic/back-to-nature movements for the past 15 years. During that time, he has advised and helped many in the art of transitioning away from mucus-forming foods. For a limited time, talk with Prof. Spira about your individual needs, challenges, and questions. Skype, telephone, or in-person consultations available! For more information, visit:

www.mucusfreelife.com/diet-coaching

WEB LINKS

Websites

mucusfreelife.com

breathairmusic.com

Facebook

Prof. Spira Fan Page: www.facebook.com/ProfessorSpira

Arnold Ehret Fan Page: www.facebook.com/arnoldehret.us

Arnold Ehret Support Group: www.facebook.com/groups/arnoldehret/

YouTube

Prof. Spira's Breathair-Vision: www.youtube.com/user/professorspira

Twitter

@profspira

@ArnoldEhret1

Visit our Bookstore to Find Books by Arnold Ehret!

www.mucusfreelife.com/storefront/

Spira is now available for mucusless diet consultations/coaching!

www.mucusfreelife.com/storefront/product/mucusless-diet-coaching/

Please Share Your Reviews!

Share your reviews and comments about this book and your experiences
with the mucusless diet on Amazon and mucusfreelife.com. Prof. Spira
would love to hear how the text has helped you.

PEACE, LOVE, AND BREATH!

Made in the USA
Monee, IL
05 October 2022